FATHERBOND

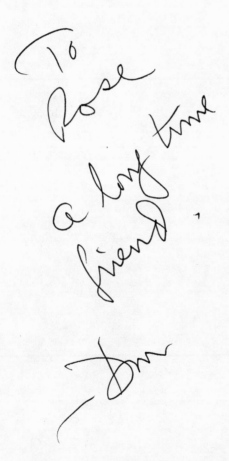

To
Rose

a long time

friend,

FATHERBOND

DON OSGOOD

Tyndale House Publishers, Inc.

WHEATON, ILLINOIS

Scripture quotations are taken from
The Holy Bible,
Revised Standard Version.

First printing, April 1989

Library of Congress Catalog Card Number 89-50087
ISBN 0-8423-0833-4
Copyright 1989 by Don Osgood
Printed in the United States of America

To our four sons—
Kevin, Jeff, Drew, and Trevor—
who bless our lives,
and to Bill and Sally Kanaga,
whose loving help eased our way

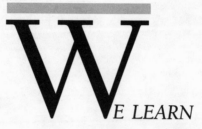

WE LEARN
from what
our fathers do
more than
from what
they say.

I DIDN'T UNDERSTAND what it really means to be a father until my son died. When the searing numbness finally wore away, I realized what I had learned.

Some say the death of your child is the most wrenching loss you can have. It is. On the brighter side, one of the most significant happenings you can have is to become a real father to your son or daughter, not just someone who sires a fragile, dependent life. Because fatherhood isn't completed at the moment of birth. For some it takes a lifetime. For me, it happened in the death of my son. For all of us it is a critical issue because of a present shortage of the kind of father I want to tell you about. As you read this, you, too, can begin to live parenthood in a new way.

I grew up to fatherhood watching the way my father died one month and the way my son died in the next. Traveling from one hospital to the other, I began to think about fatherhood in a new way. After twenty-eight years of watching our son grow into manhood, I began to *live* fatherhood in the last three months of my son's life.

Jeff changed from a handsome, successful, married man to a totally dependent, unrecognizable person whom I loved in a new way. It was all backward from the birth process, but the experience was not all tragic, as you will see. We learn far more through the painful experiences than the joy-filled times. There is no wisdom in happiness.

I cannot begin to understand the powerful impact the death of our son had on my loving wife, Joan. She and other members of our family are experiencing their own life-learning from our indescribable loss. Joan served our son in love, as did Lindy, his wife, to a depth I will never understand, though we three stood side by side for three months as we listened and spoke and prayed.

But each of us gropes for ways to express our learning. For me, speaking is healing. It is also preparing for the future, so I am speaking to you. In a way I don't understand, I may speak *for* you.

First, you must understand that being a father is not like being a mother. I'm not going to give you platitudes. The word fatherhood still means something because we have not overworked it. We have not even understood it.

Women carry the seed of motherhood within them and must react to life inside. But men must *come to fatherhood* and bring it into their lives. That is why you must hear my story with the ear of your spirit.

WHEN THE MESSAGE CAME

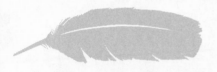

Jeff and I always had a close understanding. Perhaps that is why when the phone rang and our son Drew picked it up, he heard Jeff ask immediately, "Is Dad there?" The urgency was clear.

"I'm in the hospital, Dad," he said. "They tell me I have cancer and I won't be able to go home." Everything inside me sounded an alarm, but the male instinct said, *Reassure him.*

"Then it's good, Son," I managed to say. "They can help you best there. I'll come to the hospital right away."

Looking into Drew's eyes as I hung up, I heard him say, "He's going to die, isn't he, Dad?" Drew's penetrating insight let him know more than I was willing to let on—or believe.

"No," I said, letting my head get separated from my feelings, the way men do. "It's serious, not terminal."

On the way to the hospital, I thought a thousand things. But when I saw Jeff, we talked analytically about the kind of cancer he had.

"It may be the kind that has a 90 percent cure rate, Dad," he said. The title "Dad" felt good to me as he spoke.

"We'll know when the lab report comes back," he said, letting his scientific training encourage us, but he was watching me closely. A man with a master's degree in laser optics seeks reassurance in probability curves. That is why we were comforted when the good news came that it was the most curable cancer known.

So I left the Connecticut hospital for my father's retirement home in New York's Adirondack Mountains, where he had decided to stay instead of returning to the hospital again.

"No more hospitals. No more doctors," he said, already breathing heavily from lung cancer. Even so, he was strong in mind and heart, with fifty years of Methodist ministry and eighty-six years of wisdom behind him. I had come to a point of receiving much strength from my father.

"If I die, I die at home," he said, following his father's identical decision at age eighty-three. We learn from what our fathers do more than from what they say.

I remembered prior years when I had arrived at my parents' home, located at the edge of a forest that rolled down to the lakeside. Once, seeing my dad's joy, I said, "You like this place, don't you?" and he responded with a masculine term of endearment. "I like him," he said. He had fallen in love with the personality of the land.

fifteen

On another visit, I ran up the hillside when I arrived after I had learned he was cutting down a tree. I wanted to spy on him as he hauled the log down a snowpath, a chain in one hand and a cane in the other. There is a silent picture of fatherhood you can capture forever when no one knows you are looking.

But this time, while he was no longer strong enough to fell trees, he was strong enough to decide to die as he chose, rather than as the doctors chose.

Traveling back from the Adirondacks to Jeff's hospital, I stopped to rest at an old antique shop on the way and spotted a book printed in the 1920s by an organization called the Father and Son League. If you'd seen the book without the right timing of life and death, you'd have said it was quaint or unsophisticated. But not when you know your father is dying and your son might be.

When I showed it to Jeff, he was recovering from chemotherapy, so I asked him if he'd like me to read it to

T

HE WORD *fatherhood still means something because we have not overworked it. We have not even understood it.*

him. Sometimes a fifty-five-year-old father can read to a twenty-eight-year-old son and it's all right. Head and heart were coming together with some help from the 1920s.

That paved the way for deeper communication just a few days later when I called Jeff in the morning. His voice on the phone betrayed the special fear a battle with cancer can bring.

THE ISOLATION ROOM

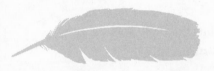

"They're moving me into the isolation room today, Dad," he said, the weakness evident in his thin voice.

I tried to use words that would reveal hope behind the clouds of Jeff's uncertainty.

"This may be a good sign, Jeff. The chemotherapy is finally working."

But here we were in the fourth week of Jeff's hospitalization with still no evidence that the cancer in his chest was easing its three-fisted grip on his heart, lungs, and thoracic duct. Now the dreaded chemotherapy had begun to kill his white blood cells, and the life struggle between the cancer, the chemotherapy, and Jeff's immune system had begun.

"I'll be there as soon as I can, Jeff," I said.

"Yes," he said, but his reply was so weak that his voice had no expression.

Racing along the interstate to the hospital, I prayed, "Let me get there in time, please."

They were just rolling Jeff's bed away as I arrived. "I'm here," I announced as brightly as I could without appearing insincere to Jeff's scientific mind.

"You'll need to wear this mask now," the nurse said. "And you'll need to scrub your hands whenever you enter the room."

As the nurses left, I realized this was a special moment of resignation—or renewal. How many times in life do you spend with your son in isolation? Will it be an imprisonment or a spiritual discovery?

The room seemed cramped, and the fresh August morning outside suddenly seemed far away. "I may be here for seven days or so," Jeff was saying, looking up at me from his shadowed bed. He had a feeding tube in his groin, a draining tube in his chest, and a colorless face. His weakness and discouragement were plain now.

The emotion was too much for the moment, but we hung on as I turned away quickly and explored the room for him, making little meaningless observations and searching for the words he needed to hear.

"Your own shower!" I commented through my sanitary mask.

"Good," he said, pretending encouragement along with me. Then the wisdom of the Lord came quietly, gracefully.

"Jeff, it's so easy for us to notice the big things in life. This may be the moment to notice the intimate attention of God in the little places." He looked at me thoughtfully, not responding, caught with the idea.

We talked then of Brother Lawrence, the French monk in the 1600s who practiced the Presence of God for thirty years in his lonely kitchen and changed the lives of uncounted people who came to listen for and observe the Presence. I read aloud some of Brother Lawrence's ancient letters, noticing now that Jeff's eyes were closed. His face looked chiseled and pale against his dark hair and full beard. I wondered, *Is this how he will look if he loses out?* But these are the fear-filled thoughts you crowd out of your mind quickly.

Then I began to realize some of the little secrets of life. This first night of isolation with Jeff was mine. The next would belong to my wife, Joan, then Jeff's wife, Lindy, then his older brother, Kevin. Kevin wanted to be a spiritual brother to Jeff so they could talk of their growing up together. This first night, Lindy, who was a nurse, thoughtfully arranged for a cot for me. And in the dark night of

*THE
quality of our
communication
depends
on finding
simple ways
to serve.*

isolation, I felt a helpless communion I couldn't explain.

My thoughts raced back over the twenty-eight years of Jeff's life to a night when I had noticed him looking out through the bars of his crib while I read a bedtime story to his older brother, Kevin, in the youth bed across the room. The next night, I had climbed into Jeff's crib, which creaked and groaned under my weight, to read the bedtime story to him.

I wondered how I could do that again in some symbolic way, now that Jeff had become a needy son again. So I touched his foot, thinking, *What can a father do for a twenty-eight-year-old son?*

Amazingly, I found that massaging the soles of his feet had a remarkable affect on his sense of comfort, and his attitude seemed to change from resignation to appreciation. I began to see that the quality of our communication depends on finding simple ways to serve. In the midst of Jeff's sedated pain, he stirred and asked thickly, "How can you love me so much, Dad?"

I listened as Jeff slept, groaning with labored breath through the night, mercifully waking only a few times. In the gray light of the early morning, I found myself sitting up, looking at Jeff silently, sensing he was awake. Then he spoke, his eyes still closed.

"Did you sleep well, Dad?"

"Yes, I did. I was very tired."

Looking at me, he said, "Maybe this is irrational, but I'm afraid of things in the early morning."

"I know, Jeff. I am, too."

"I'm afraid of things that don't make sense later in the day."

"Yes. I am, too."

"Can we pray about being afraid?"

I knew Jeff was experiencing what many people feel at 4:00 A.M., so it was easy to understand. Then a quiet, unrepeatable flow of wisdom about fear and love and life came in a soothing stream of words—a gift from the Presence in the room. We were practicing the Presence of God with our prayer, perhaps as Brother Lawrence had in the 1600s. We were letting fear flow out as love flowed in, discovering there isn't room for both.

When our words were over, Jeff asked, "Could we read a psalm now?"

"Which one?" I asked.

"Psalm 21, I think . . . or maybe that isn't the one."

The psalm was unfamiliar to both of us, but I turned to it, looking for a message for Jeff. He had breezed through life, it seemed—through a graduate degree in physics, a blossoming marriage, and a position of scientific leadership. Now, suddenly, he was reduced to frail dependence in an isolation room.

The psalm was one of King David's, written at a time when he, too, began to recognize his dependence on God. Behind the thoughts of a successful king unfolded a message for Jeff and for me; we recognized a kindred helplessness. The words of David that meant the most

I N the rising
of our sun
seen through
the narrow
windows
of our lives,
there is love,
given to fathers
and sons
as they spend
time together.

to us were these: "In thy strength the king rejoices, O Lord; and in thy help how greatly he exults. . . . He asked life of thee; thou gavest it to him. . . . Thou dost make him glad with the joy of thy presence. For the king trusts in the Lord; and through the steadfast love of the Most High he shall not be moved."

The words "The king trusts in the Lord" were especially helpful. We were learning to trust, too—not in scientific power or the modern privileges of technology contained in the beeping and humming equipment surrounding us. We saw that a physicist, too, must trust in the Lord. We had been helped along in our trust by spiritual discernment contained in the humble words of a French monk from the 1600s and in the strong words of a king in ancient Jerusalem. But we also felt an abiding Presence that had been literally prayed into the isolation room by hundreds of friends across northeast America.

The Lord's message came to us in our isolation, as it comes now to you in whatever isolation you feel in life. "You are not alone. You never were. You never shall be, because I am present in your isolation."

In the rising of the sun seen through the narrow windows of our lives, there is love, given to fathers and sons as they spend time together.

A NEW
DIAGNOSIS

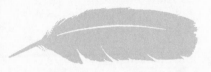

But Jeff's condition turned still worse. I was in his room when the specialist told him the original diagnosis had been wrong. The specialist was remarkably open, as doctors have become through necessity. I don't envy them at times like these.

"The diagnosis was wrong," she said. "It looked like another form of cancer."

"What's the recovery rate of this cancer?" Jeff asked, calling on his trust in such things as probability and data analysis.

There was a sophisticated pause, then an even-voiced report. "It would have been 50 percent if the doctors had diagnosed it correctly five weeks ago. Now it's 30 percent."

Even the stillness in the room was stunning. It was as though a strong young tree were falling silently in the woods.

With several people standing around, how do fathers and sons speak in such a moment? Lindy handled this as she did everything—in a brave and loving way. So did my wife, Joan. But since our consideration is about fathers and sons, I want to confine my story to what happened to Jeff and me.

Jeff looked at me, speechless. A question was forming in his eyes. It was a long and unflinching look as he searched for an answer in my eyes, and I marveled at his control. He didn't need to speak.

I knew I was to be a father in what I did next. But how do you stop a tree from falling?

"What are our options, doctor?" I asked.

It was the only way I knew to get through a moment that no one ever wants to have. In such a time, your instinct says, *Get into possibilities. Get into solutions. Get out of this.* It was the only way to move through an impossible moment.

Mercifully, everyone was quickly gone but Jeff and me; Lindy cried in another room. Jeff said, "For the first time in my life, I feel that a year from now I won't be alive."

"Maybe not," I said, realizing this was a moment of honesty, yet wishing I could change what was happening.

"I know I won't ever suffer as much as our Lord," he said surprising me.

I wondered. *Do you speak of death to your son? What gives him strength? What brings you closer? What fosters real fatherhood?* Then the gift of wisdom came.

"Whether you live or die, Jeff, God will not leave you."

"Yes," he said, looking at me.

"He loves you either way."

thirty-three

"Yes, either way."

Our strength to move through this moment was born in honesty. Honesty is reassuring. Protective white lies ultimately bottle up your fear.

Yet even more than honesty was needed now. Strangely, it was a comfort to both of us to turn *to* something . . . to anything that seemed stronger than death. We were a father and a son looking at death together and hooking up with the Author of fatherhood. We were tapping the same strength that God had when his Son was facing death.

But in a quiet meditation room moments later, I cried with the great, heaving sobs of human grief that come from down so deep within you that all your body cries. It seemed the young tree had crashed without a roar, yet I had to break the prison of stillness. Men must cry somewhere.

This was the son I had climbed in the crib with to read a bedtime story. The

IT WAS
as though
a strong
young tree
were falling
silently
in the woods. . . .
But how
do you stop
a tree
from falling?

one who leaned his head against my shoulder as I read. But God speaks in his silent language in the crisis times.

"He will be all right. He won't die yet."

NEW YORK CITY

So we moved Jeff from Connecticut to the best cancer hospital we could find in New York. Even though the ambulance lost its way, we were filled with new hope as Jeff finally arrived. Looking into his eyes as he lay beside an East River view he couldn't see, I said, "We're moving into the city to be here with you. We're changing our entire life schedule for you, Jeff. You won't be alone."

With the support of his wife and his mother by his side, I was able to travel back to my father, dying now in the Adirondacks. And I learned with him how to speak of dying.

"I want to go soon," my father said, looking shockingly thin already, laboring to breathe but looking me straight in the eye.

There is a way to respond to an unspoken request of drawing a curtain over your feelings—and your eyes. Doctors know how to do this, I learned. But the professional look is just a look—uncommitted, unrevealing, just standing by. That's not being a father or being a son. I had to learn what it is to be a real son and a real father at the same time. They go together, and I found that your look at such a time must be a look of commitment and love that looks straight into the heart.

Then my father said, "I want you to pray with me that I will go quickly. I'm ready to go. There's a better place ahead for me."

It had never occurred to me that my father would require me to enter into an agreement about his death. It was a remarkable preparation for me from a dying father who was including me in a pact—and in a final ministry.

"Yes," I said, and I prayed with him on the spot. "Father," I said, thinking

I WAS
learning
a way
to get ready
for the future
by living
in the present.
We must
get out of
the future.

upward, "Please . . ." and I paused, caught momentarily in emotion.

Saying please is not begging; it is showing respect. It is what a son says when he knows his father can hear, and I knew two fathers were listening.

"Dad wants to die and I . . . agree."

There was a curious bond of freedom and love between three fathers in that moment—an unusual fatherbond. I was learning a way to get ready for the future by living in the present. We must get out of the future.

Returning from my father's mountain retreat to Manhattan's rushing streets, I now began to pray in a way I had never prayed, walking with my son and wife and daughter-in-law down the hospital corridors. We trailed the intravenous rig along on little wheels through the halls. We read by Jeff's bed, played Ping-Pong in the recreation room, and repeated Scriptures pinned all over the walls by Jeff's wife. We prayed as the early disciples prayed, and hospital employees came in to feel the strong new Presence in the room. It spread out into the hallways as we walked, and it brought in more hospital employees and more friends with strong faith and powerful prayers.

But up in the Adirondack wilderness, my father was failing fast. So I prepared to leave, and Jeff said, as he had increasingly, "Tell him I know what he's going through."

A strong identification had developed between the two bedridden men. By telephone and messenger they kept in touch.

"How's Jeff?" my father would ask each time I arrived. And I would say, "He's taking life a day at a time. He wants you to know he's with you."

"Tell him I'm praying for him," my father would say. But not this time. He couldn't talk.

THE SILENT LANGUAGE

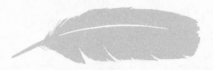

The silent language of a father is heart-winning. Standing by the foot of my father's bed, I saw him looking at me quietly as he raised his hand with special strength and blew a kiss at me. He was saying good-bye in the only way he knew how, and I spoke my thanks. Then, wanting to be a help, I gave him the only bath I ever gave my father.

I had learned much about serving someone you love. To serve as a father and a son is a part of the silent language of love you must learn if you are to become a real father. To be a real father you must become a real son. And sometimes in silent service you can be more overt than in speaking. So I began to look for added ways to be of service to my son Jeff when I returned.

But before I returned, my father died. Trevor, our youngest son, was there with me when I went outside—"for a little fresh air," I said. He sensitively came along and gave me a hug in the dark outdoors while the deep, dry sobs came. In tough times fathers and sons need to be together. Being there, however outward or passive you are, is a strong sign to both.

Later, I walked out alone at midnight to the town dock and stood looking into the blackness of the lake and the clear sky, pinpointed with millions of star lights. I called out into the dark lake and dark sky, "Dad! Dad!" But the stars didn't move.

Steam rose from far out on the lake, giving off its warmth to the cold sky. I remembered my father saying, "I'm going to take a lot of trips up there." And I wondered at his journey now as I looked up at the vast quietness.

Then I noticed something around me. The evaporation of the lake was blowing softly by me and I was immersed in it, suddenly moved by a Presence. Looking up, I recognized the silent language of God and felt included again in the bond. But in a moment I looked down at the water again, and the thin clouds of steam were surprisingly far out on the lake. I was standing alone, seemingly unprotected but now strangely comforted, at the end of the town dock—at the end of civilization.

I had wondered what it would be like with my father gone. I had assumed there would be a moment of stepping into his leadership role, but I had not guessed the moment would be so dark or so lonely.

To grow up to fatherhood, you must step out of self-preoccupation into the strength of comforting your mother. A powerful, spiritual law of the universe states that with each death is born new life, a new growth, a new acceptance that grief can be channeled into life by helping someone close to you. To grow up to fatherhood, you must look up and out to others, not just within.

When you imagine the black night is not really a universe populated by a million distant stars, but is a huge black umbrella with a million pinpoints punched through to reveal one great Light behind it, that helps you hold an earthly umbrella over your mother beside a rain-soaked grave the next day. It is a gift to serve, and that is what mature fathers and sons must do.

In the rain that day, surprisingly, was extraordinary triumph. The largest funeral in many years in that lakeside town brought together forty-one ministers who sang a song of praise. Somehow it became a graduation day for my father—and for me. I had agreed in advance to let him go.

So I returned again to be a father to Jeff, lying still on his bed in Manhattan beside the slow-flowing East River. For Jeff, life was ebbing away like the waters of the East River as they flowed toward the sea.

THE black night
is not really
a universe
populated
by a million
distant stars,
but a huge
black umbrella
with a million
pinpoints
punched through
it. . . .

He had received a severe setback while I was gone. He had hovered at the point of death while my father died, and I, mercifully, had not known. Punched now with many operations, fevered by the battering of chemotherapy, none of his wavy black hair left, he asked, "How was Gramps?"

"It was all right, Jeff."

"Did he have a hard time breathing?"

"Yes. But he saw something, Jeff."

We never spoke of my father again. There was too much happening with Jeff. The lung cancer miraculously shrank and finally vanished, but the battle scars were now too deep for recovery. The cure would become the cause of death.

In the meantime, chemotherapy would make Jeff lose his senses temporarily. Our phone rang in the Manhattan apartment at 3:00 A.M. one night, and Jeff asked for me. While he loved and trusted his wife and his mother, I think it must have been our experience in the isolation room that made him ask for me.

ONE REALITY

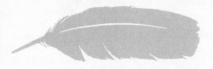

"I had to talk with you, Dad. The walls were dissolving right in front of my eyes. The molecules in the bed were separating and I could see them separating. Everything was moving and nothing was firm and I had to talk with you."

"I know, Son," I said, but I couldn't really know. I only knew he was in trouble and I was to listen.

". . . and there were strange creatures creeping over my skin," he was saying.

Twenty-nine years old now, with a hospital birthday behind him, Jeff was trying not to be destroyed by the terrifying prospect of losing his sanity. He was methodically using his scientific training to describe everything so he could master his fear. In such times, the test of real fatherhood is not to try to be the ultimate father, but to point to the real One from whom reality comes— even in the middle of living chemical nightmares.

"There is only one reality, Jeff," I said, not knowing exactly what I was going to say next.

But I was finding that we become real fathers when we recognize our strength is in reaching into the real Father's wisdom. *Seeing Jesus* provided the visual strength to make my prayer cut through the chemical power warping Jeff's mind. Since no one has seen God, we have been left a clear picture of Jesus. So I prayed that Jeff would see a real Jesus instead of creatures and dissolving walls.

Cancer, this indescribable illness, is a terror. There is a sense of evil in it as it grows inside you, living off your body, trying to take your life. It signifies a struggle between good and evil, and at times the chemical cure breaks your ability to see good. You literally see a fright-filled, unimaginable world.

So Jesus, the Presence sent so we could see strength in our time of weakness, allowed me to be a leader *to* the Strength when I couldn't be the source of strength myself. Fathers must be spiritual leaders but must not try to be God. And fathers can describe the way to God's strength only as they learn to see it with faith.

Fear is the special tool of Satan that blinds our vision to the God-strength that is available even when we are deathly afraid. Faith is the opposite of fear and conquers it.

When there isn't enough faith in just one of us, there is enough in two. So Jeff and I conquered our fear by seeing Jesus as we prayed. And the next morning, a rested Jeff said, "Thanks. I went to sleep last night when I hung up."

I began to see an unusual spiritual sense growing stronger in Jeff. It had been there all along as we recognized together the simple-seeming gifts we share in life—the texture of grass and the sound of fresh wind blowing among the trees.

Now, as Jeff lost the privileges of open windows and of nature's textures—even of eating—I began to pray at meals with new appreciation for simple joys. *Thank you, Lord, for the feel of the wind against my face.* Just because there is so much of it, air is no less a miracle. We can gulp huge lung-fulls of it, and its supply never ends. It is a lifetime gift we spend most of our lives overlooking.

But not Jeff. It was my bittersweet privilege to be with him on his last night of breathing by himself. You realize how strong our love for air is when you see your son suddenly lose it.

We were alone that night for a reason I did not know in advance. I had felt I should stay overnight again with Jeff, on the floor beside his bed, just to be there. Suddenly, about midnight, he could hardly breathe.

THE TEST
of real
fatherhood
is not to try
to be the
ultimate father,
but to point
to the real One
from whom
reality comes.

"Something's . . . gone . . . wrong," he said between labored breaths. The nurse gave him something and assured us it would resolve his discomfort in breathing.

For forty-five minutes Jeff fought for air, holding his arms out to the railings to expand his lungs. Finally, I realized the nurse's repeated assurances were faulty. I saw Jeff looking at me with pleading eyes that tore me inside. When I found the intern, he gave Jeff 100 percent oxygen, but outside the room he cautioned me.

"I can't keep him on 100 percent oxygen for long. He will be damaged by it." Then he looked at me and said, "Anything can happen, you know."

I knew.

For a brief moment, I was angry. Later, my minister asked me if I was angry at God, and I said yes. Then began the long road to healing and the deep under-standing that being honest about anger is the underlying requirement for healing of any loss. But you don't have time to recognize anger when your son may be dying.

I went back to Jeff, who was breathing in precious oxygen. He said, "Dad, will you pray with me?"

Standing by Jeff's bed now, after three months of standing by, I had no more words to pray. We had prayed all the ways we knew how to pray, as had hundreds of people across America. But now the doctors were saying that a breathing machine was the only hope. What does a father do when his son agrees to go on a breathing machine and knows more than you do about what that means?

"We will need sign language, Dad."

"All right."

"This means I'm OK and this means I'm not," he said, gesturing in the air.

"Yes," I said, looking closely at his sign language.

"This means 'Lindy' and this means 'Dad' and this means 'Mom.'"

Now, standing by his bed to pray, I knew words were not sufficient after just discussing sign language. All I could do was recognize that I had no power at all. Words of encouragement were empty. There was only one word that seemed powerful enough.

"Jesus," I said. And then I reverted to the memorized songs I had learned when I was a boy at home in a Methodist parsonage.

"Jesus . . . is the sweetest name I know," I said. "I see you, Jesus. *We see you, Jesus.*"

I was consciously turning to someone who knew more than I did about suffering, to the one whom my father had turned to and his father had turned to. Both had been ministers. Both died of cancer in their beds at home and must have seen the same power I was seeing now in my prayer. Unless fathers *see* the way, they have less power to be strong fathers in the ultimate crises of life.

THE PRESENCE

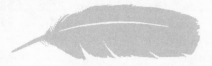

I felt someone come up behind me and over to Jeff, lying at my left. I was so startled at the swiftness of the person who had come in that I looked to Jeff's side but, amazingly, I saw no one. Jeff was looking at me and must have seen my look of dismay. In my confusion at not seeing the reality of the Presence there, I couldn't look any longer and bowed my head silently, not noticing that Jeff had become someone different.

Then I felt Jeff's fingers reaching mine and weakly squeezing them.

He was comforting me.

"Will you stand beside me, Dad, while I pray?" It was a calm, loving voice I heard, and I moved closer to listen. I was about to experience the same bond God had created with my father and me, this time with my son.

"Dear Lord," he whispered, his hand rising up as though on a witness stand. It was the pact again.

"Help me to stand by you, Lord, *whatever happens.*"

I could not speak. My son was now stronger than I.

Finally, exhausted, I said, "I'll just lie here beside your bed so I'll be ready . . . when the doctor comes."

"Yes," he said. "You rest now, Dad."

When they came for Jeff, I followed beside him, right up to the swinging doors of the intensive care room. As the doors swung open, I called after him loudly, "I'll be right here, Jeff. I'll be in there as soon as they let me."

Lying on the floor outside the doors, I waited, only half realizing the miracle of growth that had been taking place in Jeff. It is the privilege and the responsibility of a father to recognize the quiet miracles when they occur, but it takes time at first. Stretched out on the floor in the middle of the night, you pray for one miracle, while often another far deeper miracle is happening.

When the nurse came to me and said, "You can come in now. He's awake," I hurried in and saw the big tube down Jeff's throat and recognized the pain as the nurse vacuumed out the residue from his lungs. The tube was so large.

"Jeff," I said. He coughed.

"Jeff, I'm here."

I desperately wanted him to hear me. I put my hand on his forehead to bless him with my prayer.

"Jesus is here, Jeff. I see you, Jesus," I said, and Jeff instantly relaxed into a deep sleep from which he never moved.

We were never able to use our sign language. So I spoke to Jeff for a week, as we all did. I reached the point of imagining Jeff's prayer and speaking it for him. I became his tongue. His silent language was expressed in an occasional counter breath as he fought the machine. It was the only way he could communicate, according to the doctors.

But in all of this, I was learning the silent language of God, as all fathers can in time. We sense a little of this silent language when fishing or walking along a beach, but this was in the hospital, *in the Presence*. Brother Lawrence felt this Presence, and I felt it again with Jeff.

THE GIFT OF
THE BLESSING

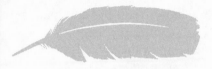

It is the gift of fathers to feel the Presence of God and to bless their children with it. Placing your hand on your son's or daughter's head when you pray is a special privilege that all fathers have, whether it is each night at bedtime for young children or in the hospital when they are sick or at their wedding. It is your privilege to bless, handed down from Old Testament days. In so doing, you prepare your son or daughter for the Presence of God.

Then it is your equal responsibility to step aside and let God be the father to your child. After all is said, you must let your son or daughter transfer trust in you to trust in the real Source of fatherhood. That is your role in parental blessing—to believe that God is not only your strength but also your son's or daughter's strength.

We must let go willingly. But it is so hard to let go until you finally see that holding on is standing in the way of the truth that sets us free. God was and is and will be our Father . . . especially in the unbearable times. When you give back to God your child in the final crisis of life, you have not lost him, just as God, in giving you a child, has not lost him. You must see God in everything.

Months later, while still recovering from Jeff's death, I attended the National Prayer Breakfast, a daylong event held in Washington, D.C., along with thousands of others, including the president. A little-known leader of one of the workshops there unlocked a powerful insight for me. He said, "When you look into the eyes of someone who is suffering, Jesus looks back at you." I was struck with this statement, knowing then that somehow Jesus was entering in a

I

T IS the
gift of fathers
to feel the
Presence of God
and to bless
their children
with it.

more powerful way into Jeff when I felt the Presence move behind me to Jeff's side.

As fathers, we have a special power to call on this strength for our children. When we fix our eyes on the Christ and call his name, we receive all the power of God it is possible for us to receive. And it spills over into family members so they can receive it and become strong beyond imagination. Ultimately, fathers must *stand by* to let this force flow. In stepping aside willingly, having served all we can, only then do we experience fatherhood, perhaps in the way God experienced a new phase of fatherhood when he let Jesus die.

THROUGH A MOVING WINDOW

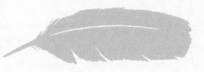

Months later, I began to enter the world of business again, having learned to look at life more clearly, as though looking through a moving window.

I had caught an early train from Connecticut to Wilmington, Delaware, one morning. Gliding quietly past Manhattan, shining yellow in the early morning sun as it waited for the day's swarming commuters, my train arched away, across the East River. I could see the inspiring parade of buildings, looking as though they had marched up the length of Manhattan and now stood at parade rest, mute and glorious in the sun.

My special knowledge of a certain building pulled my eyes unwillingly toward Midtown and the familiar outline of a soaring hospital, hiding behind it the smaller hospital where my son had died.

There will always be a spiritual tug when I see that place, alive then with confident-faced doctors, comprising the best that a world of cancer fighters could muster. But they later stood by, powerless and mask-like, as Jeff's spirit went quietly up through the floors, leaving his battle for life behind.

Now the hospital was insignificant, impossible to spot, buried among the rise and sweep of Manhattan's buildings as they stretched across my train window like some cinema scene. Did God really intend that many buildings on one island?

Earlier, on a recovery trip to Venice, I had marvelled when I looked beyond masterpiece structures of ancient builders to the real miracles walking by. Did God intend people to walk by buildings in that much awe of man's creation?

But as I looked at the sweep of Manhattan, perspective came. I saw the little size of that once-important hospital—and the relative smallness of all Manhattan—compared to the depth and expanse of the brilliant blue ocean of air over it. I began to see that we live at the bottom of this ocean, pushing priceless air around between us as we move. When Jeff died, he came up through the hospital floors to the top of our ocean—came up, not for air, but to fill his lungs with freedom. Maybe that's why I felt the inexplicable tugging upward as I had stood over Jeff's bed, knowing he was above, not below me.

Suddenly, I caught a faint glimpse of another world, as though someone had tilted the train window to reflect a far different place in the Adirondacks, where my father had died only a month before Jeff.

The glimpse of the Adirondacks, superimposed over Manhattan, showed a towering tumble of mountains and huge, numberless evergreen trees dipping their roots in the water of the Hudson while it was still the clean water of the North River flowing down toward Manhattan.

While the mountain waters streamed down, these giant evergreens had climbed their way up the mountains with glacial slowness, dropping their seeds generation by generation. They now stood tiptoe atop the mountains, reaching up yet further into the same blue ocean of air.

When my father died in his little red-roofed retirement cottage by the lake, tucked in the shadow of one of those ancient mountains, surrounded by great evergreens marching on in generations, I realized he had only the attic to rise through before hitting the freedom of the open air.

Swiftly and quietly, he had become a part of the mountain's mute history. I was left as seed for another time, beginning to accept that God allows

GOD doesn't
look down on us
or through a
windowpane
at us.
Instead,
he sits
in the seat
beside us.

great trees to fall and other trees to take their place on the mountain.

All of that grandeur shadowed the picture in the moving pane. At that moment, looking at Manhattan slide by my train window, I saw the spiritual picture I was supposed to see. These giant cities and awesome mountains we wind our way through are only the *places* God loves, some built by him, some by us. What he is really looking at is us. The real miracles swarm their way to work and home, not noticing how *little* the cities and mountains are compared to the blue ocean they are submerged in. I couldn't see anyone looking down on Manhattan, but I could sense the spiritual vision of a God who watches over teeming cities and lonely mountains to find someone who will look up and say, "I see You."

While we watch passively through our framed windowpanes on life trains that rush us through our schedules for a mere twenty-nine or eighty-six years—it matters little the length—we have a brief opportunity to sense the majesty of why God set it all in motion in the first place. At least for mutual recognition, not just for a view through a one-way mirror of some kind.

But can you see God even when you can't see the blue? When you are plunged into darkness?

My train looped back toward the city, rushing at it with determination until we were swallowed up in the darkness of a tunnel. Here, underground, with some people leaving the train before others boarded for Washington and other seemingly important destinations, the engine was unhooked, plunging the cars into darkness. The view through my window was gray and black.

Am I looking through the dimness now to find him? Is his eye on me? Is he watching, not just an Adirondack attic away or twenty hospital floors away, but through the black earth to me?

I sensed an answer. In the transition from one perspective to another, from one life to another, God doesn't look down on us or through a windowpane at us. Instead, he sits in the seat beside us, saying, "I've been here with you, watching the whole scene through your eyes. Someday I'll give you a chance to see it through mine. And when you find it hard to swim up through the ocean, I will breathe for you, through your lungs. But for now, I want you to work with me, on this train."

Then that's how it was with Jeff, I thought. *That's how it's been all along. And that's how it will be!* Someday I'll say:

Good-bye, windowpanes.
Good-bye, labored lungs.
Hello, freedom.

But all in good patience.
All in good time.

Now I've got work to do
With the person
Sitting next to me.

God doesn't enjoy
Our passive peeking
Through little windows.

Too many fathers have done that
For too long.

Good-bye, Dad. Good-bye, Son.
Hello, Brother.

We grow up to fatherhood by being
brothers. Now. You and I.